NATURAL REMEDIES FOR HEART DISEASES MANAGEMENT

The Proven Ways To Treat Disease At Home

TERESA E. LUNA

Table of Contents:

The introduction of natural remedies for heart disease management

Many people are afflicted by heart disease, which is a frequent and dangerous health problem. Although traditional therapies like medicine and surgery can be successful in managing cardiac disease, there are also some natural approaches that can. Included in these remedies are:

lifestyle modifications For good heart health, one should adopt a balanced diet, engage in regular exercise, give up smoking, and control stress.

Supplements: It has been demonstrated that supplements including omega-3 fatty acids, coenzyme Q10, and magnesium can help control heart disease.

Herbs: Research has demonstrated the positive effects of several herbs, including hawthorn, ginger, and garlic, on heart health.

Acupuncture: Research on this traditional Chinese medicine has shown that it can help lower blood pressure and increase circulation, all of which are crucial for heart health.

The use of natural remedies should not be considered a substitute for medical care, it is crucial to remember. Before attempting any new remedies or treatments, it is always advisable to speak with your doctor.

heart disease explanation

The phrase "heart disease" is used to refer broadly to a number of illnesses that have an impact on the heart and blood vessels. It can be used to describe illnesses that affect the heart muscle, like coronary artery disease and heart attacks, as well as illnesses that affect the blood arteries that lead to and from the heart, like atherosclerosis and stroke. Heart disease is the world's largest cause of death and disability, and it's frequently linked to things like high blood pressure, high cholesterol, smoking, and a sedentary lifestyle.

Chest pain, shortness of breath, heart palpitations, and weariness are just a few of the symptoms of heart disease that can manifest in many ways. While some types of heart disease are acquired by lifestyle choices and age, others are genetic.

Heart disease is accompanied by a number of risk factors, such as:

Age: Growing older raises your risk of developing heart disease.

Family history: Your risk is higher if you have heart disease in your family.

Smoking: Smoking harms blood vessels and the heart, raising the risk of heart disease.

High blood pressure: High blood pressure puts extra strain on the heart and blood vessels and can cause heart disease.

Heart disease can result from fatty deposits accumulating in the blood arteries due to high cholesterol levels.

Sedentary behavior: Heart disease risk can rise with inactivity.

Making good lifestyle decisions, including eating a balanced diet, exercising frequently, giving up smoking, and managing stress, are important for both preventing and treating heart disease. To help control heart disease, a doctor could also suggest certain medications and treatments.

Information about heart disease prevalence
Millions of people around the world are impacted by heart disease, a serious public health concern. Heart disease, which claims more than 17 million lives annually, is the leading cause of mortality worldwide, according to the World Health Organization (WHO). With heart disease accounting for 1 in every 4 fatalities in the US, it is the most common cause of death.

Various factors, including age, gender, and location, affect the prevalence of heart disease. The largest risk for getting heart disease is often found in men and women over 65. Due to elements including poor diets and sedentary lifestyles, those who reside in high-income nations are also more at risk.

It's crucial to remember that many heart disease instances can be avoided with lifestyle modifications, early detection, and treatment. People can dramatically lower their risk of developing heart disease by eating healthily, exercising frequently, and managing risk factors including high blood pressure and cholesterol.

Reducing Heart Disease Risk Through Lifestyle Changes

The management of cardiac disease depends heavily on changes in lifestyle. The following adjustments can promote heart health and lower the chance of developing heart disease:

Routine exercise On most days of the week, aim for at least 30 minutes of moderate exercise, such as brisk walking.

Consume a balanced diet Put an emphasis on consuming complete foods, such as fresh produce, whole grains, and lean protein. Reduce your intake of processed food and items high in saturated and trans fats.

Reduce your risk of heart disease by quitting smoking. The heart's health can be considerably improved by quitting smoking.

Reduce alcohol consumption: Drinking too much can raise blood pressure and increase the risk of heart disease.

Manage your stress: Prolonged stress can raise your risk of developing heart disease. Find healthy stress-reduction techniques, such as exercise, meditation, or chatting to a close friend.

Keep a healthy weight: Heart disease is more likely in people who are overweight or obese. Through nutrition and exercise, try to keep a healthy weight.

Reduce cholesterol and blood pressure: Heart disease is significantly increased by high cholesterol and blood pressure. These risk factors can be reduced with the aid of medications and lifestyle modifications.

Since every patient has a different scenario, it is crucial to consult a doctor to decide the best course of action for managing heart disease. Reducing the risk of heart disease and enhancing general health and wellbeing can be accomplished by changing one's lifestyle.

Habits of a Healthy Diet

In controlling cardiac disease, healthy dietary practices are crucial. Here are some essential pointers for keeping up a heart-healthy diet:

Consume a variety of fruits and vegetables: Per day, try to eat at least 5 servings of fruits and vegetables.

Select whole grains: Rather than choosing refined, processed grains, choose whole-grain bread, rice, and pasta.

Utilize lean protein: Select lean protein sources over fatty meat cuts, such as fish, poultry, and lentils.

Avoid saturated and trans fats: Steer clear of meals high in trans and saturated fats including butter, fatty meats, and baked pastries.

Cut back on salt intake: High salt intake raises blood pressure and raises the chance of developing heart disease. Try to keep your daily sodium intake to no more than 2,300 mg.

Increase your consumption of fiber to protect your heart and assist lower cholesterol levels. Fruits and vegetables, whole grains, legumes, and veggies are excellent sources of fiber.

Include foods high in heart-healthy fats, such as nuts, seeds, and oily salmon, in your diet.

Everyone has different demands, therefore it's crucial to consult a doctor or a qualified dietitian when deciding on the optimal diet to manage heart disease. Making healthy eating a top priority can lower the risk of heart disease and enhance general health and wellbeing.

A heart-healthy diet includes both decreasing toxic substances and incorporating healthy foods. Here are some more recommendations for eating a heart-healthy diet:

Consume fish at least twice every week: Omega-3 fatty acids are abundant in fish, especially fatty fish like salmon, and they have been shown to lower inflammation and promote heart health.

Be sure to eat nuts and seeds: Almonds, walnuts, and flaxseeds are just a few of the nuts and seeds that are high in fiber, protein, and heart-healthy unsaturated fats.

Select wholesome oils: Avoid saturated and trans fats by using healthy oils like avocado and olive oil.

Reduce additional sugars: Heart disease risk has been linked to excessive added sugar consumption. Try to keep your intake of added sugars to a minimum by avoiding sugary beverages and opting for whole fruits over fruit juice or sweets.

Avoid processed foods since they frequently contain harmful fats, salt, and added sugars and can raise your risk of developing heart disease. In every case, opt for whole, unprocessed foods.

Take a look at plant-based diets: Studies have indicated that eating a vegetarian or vegan diet can enhance heart health and lower your chance of developing heart disease.

It's crucial to keep in mind that everyone has different needs, so finding the ideal nutritional strategy for controlling heart disease requires consultation with a doctor or registered dietitian. An important factor in lowering the risk of heart disease and enhancing general health and wellbeing is establishing heart-healthy eating habits.

Regular Exercise

The management of heart disease and lowering the risk of heart disease depend on regular exercise. Here are some pointers for adding fitness to your schedule:

Attempt to engage in moderate-intensity exercise most days of the week for at least 30 minutes: This can involve exercises like cycling, swimming, or brisk walking.

Utilize strength training By increasing muscle mass and decreasing body fat, strength training can aid to enhance heart health.

Find a hobby you like: Pick an activity you enjoy doing because it will be simpler to stick to a schedule.

Give it high priority: Try to schedule your workouts like any other appointment to give them prominence in your daily routine.

Make it a social activity: Working out with friends or family can make it more fun. Consider signing up for a leisure sports league or a group exercise class.

Increase intensity gradually: As your fitness level rises, start with moderate-intensity exercise and progressively increase it.

Before beginning a new workout regimen, it's crucial to consult a doctor, especially if you have any underlying medical issues. Regular exercise can lower the risk of heart disease and enhance heart health.

Numerous advantages to treating heart disease and enhancing heart health can be derived from regular exercise. Here are a few more advantages of frequent exercise:

Lowers blood pressure: By increasing blood flow and lowering stress levels, exercise can help lower blood pressure.

Increases "good" (HDL) cholesterol and decreases "bad" (LDL) cholesterol, improving cholesterol levels. Regular exercise has been found to have this effect.

Increases heart health: Strengthening the heart muscle and lowering the risk of heart disease are two ways that regular exercise can assist enhance heart health.

Exercise can help you maintain a healthy weight, which is vital for lowering your chance of developing heart disease.

Elevated energy levels make it easier to maintain an active lifestyle. Regular exercise can elevate energy levels and prevent weariness.

Exercise has been demonstrated to lower stress and enhance mental wellness, which can be advantageous for heart health.

Finding an exercise regimen that works for you is crucial, as is progressively increasing your intensity as your fitness level rises. A balanced diet, regular exercise, and other lifestyle modifications can all have a big impact on managing heart disease and lowering the chance of developing it.

Limiting alcohol consumption and giving up smoking

Limiting alcohol use and giving up smoking are two crucial lifestyle adjustments for controlling heart disease and lowering the risk of developing it.

Giving up smoking: Smoking is a significant contributor to the development of heart disease and is linked to a number of health issues, such as an increased risk of heart attack, stroke, and lung cancer. One of the most crucial things you can do for your heart health is to stop smoking.

limiting alcohol consumption Heart disease risk has been linked to excessive alcohol drinking. To lower the risk of heart disease, alcohol use should be kept to a minimum. For women, the American Heart Association advises limiting alcohol consumption to one drink per day, while for men, the recommendation is two drinks per day.

Making lifestyle adjustments, such as giving up smoking and consuming less alcohol, can significantly lower your chance of developing heart disease and improve your heart health. Working with a doctor to choose the best course of action for controlling heart disease and changing your lifestyle is crucial.

Here are some other ideas for cutting back on drinking and quitting smoking:
Smoking cessation: Although it can be difficult, there are numerous options available to help you stop, such as counseling, support groups, and nicotine replacement treatment. Your doctor can advise you on the most effective method for stopping smoking.
advantages of giving up smoking Your heart health can benefit from quitting smoking in a variety of ways, including decreased risk of heart attack and stroke, improved circulation, and decreased stress.
limiting alcohol consumption Your heart health can benefit from limiting alcohol consumption in a variety of ways, including decreased risk of heart disease, improved cholesterol levels, and decreased blood pressure.

Risks of binge drinking alcohol: Numerous health issues, such as liver disease, cancer, and heart disease, have been related to excessive alcohol use. In order to lower the danger of these health issues, alcohol consumption should be kept to a minimum.

There are several ways to control your alcohol use, such as by establishing boundaries for yourself, refraining from drinking in public, and engaging in non-alcohol-related activities.

Both giving up smoking and consuming less alcohol are crucial measures in controlling heart disease and lowering the chance of developing it. Working with a doctor to choose the best course of action for changing your lifestyle and enhancing your heart health is crucial.

Here are some additional suggestions for giving up smoking and consuming less alcohol in addition to the advantages and methods already mentioned:

Avoiding triggers, such as being around smokers or specific events that make you want to smoke, can help you stop smoking. Alternate methods of stress management, such as exercise or deep breathing, can also be used.

Limiting alcohol consumption: You might try mixing alcoholic beverages with non-alcoholic ones, like water or juice, to assist reduce your alcohol consumption. You can also look for non-alcohol alternatives for socializing and having fun.

Support is crucial because: Although giving up smoking and consuming alcohol in moderation might be difficult, having support from loved ones, friends, and medical professionals can go a long way. Working with a counselor or joining a support group might also be beneficial.

implementing moderate change It might be difficult to abruptly alter your way of life, such as giving up smoking or consuming less alcohol. Making changes gradually might simplify the process and help you stay to your objectives.

Identifying triggers You can avoid your triggers and find it simpler to stop or reduce your consumption if you are aware of them.

Relapse prevention: It's common to experience setbacks when trying to quit smoking or reduce alcohol consumption, but it's crucial to stay dedicated to your goals and avoid relapses.

Making lifestyle adjustments, including giving up smoking and drinking less alcohol, can significantly improve heart health and lower the risk of heart disease. It's crucial to seek support as needed and consult a doctor to decide the best course of action for making adjustments.

Stress Management Techniques

Techniques for controlling stress are crucial for treating cardiac disease and lowering the chance of developing it. Here are a few typical stress-reduction methods:

Exercise: Regular exercise can strengthen the heart and lower stress levels.

Exercises that include deep breathing, such as controlled breathing or meditation, can lower stress and enhance heart health.

Exercises that promote relaxation: Exercises that promote relaxation, like yoga or progressive muscle relaxation, can help lower stress and strengthen the heart.
Time management: By lowering the sense of overburden, effective time management can help lower stress levels.
Cognitive-behavioral therapy (CBT): CBT is a sort of treatment that can assist people in altering stress-inducing thoughts and actions.
Support from friends and family: Discussing your stress with friends and family can help you feel less stressed and have better heart health.
Laughter: Having fun and finding humor in life helps lower stress levels and strengthen the heart.
Techniques for controlling stress can be very helpful in treating heart disease and

lowering the chance of developing it. It's crucial to get support when necessary and consult a doctor to find the appropriate stress management strategy.

There are several methods for controlling stress; some of the most popular ones are as follows:

Exercise: Regular exercise can help lower stress and enhance mental health.

The techniques of mindfulness and meditation can assist to clear the mind and lessen tension and anxiety.

Deep breathing: Taking long, leisurely breaths helps soothe the body and mind and help lower heart rate.

Time management: Setting priorities and creating lists of things to do can help people feel less overwhelmed.

Social support: Having a sense of community and lowering stress can be achieved by hanging out with friends and family or joining a support group.

Techniques for relaxation: Yoga, tai chi, or listening to music can all be used to calm the body and mind.

Healthy living practices: Keeping a balanced diet, getting adequate sleep, abstaining from drugs, and drinking in moderation can all assist to enhance general wellbeing and lower stress.

It's critical to identify the methods that suit you best and incorporate them into your everyday practice.

Sure! I'd be pleased to go into further detail about each of the stress-reduction methods I mentioned earlier:

Exercise: Studies have shown that engaging in regular physical activity can assist to reduce stress and anxiety as well as mood and general mental health. Simple forms of exercise include going for a brisk walk, a run, or joining a fitness class. The goal is to incorporate exercise into your daily routine on a regular basis.

Mindfulness and meditation Focusing on the present moment and becoming aware of your thoughts, feelings, and bodily sensations are key components of these techniques. They can do this by encouraging relaxation, elevating mood, and enhancing feelings of inner peace, which can all assist to lessen stress and anxiety. Yoga, guided meditations, mindfulness applications, and other techniques can all be used to develop mindfulness and meditation.

Deep breathing: Managing stress by taking calm, deep breaths is easy but beneficial. It has been demonstrated that using this technique will assist lower heart rate, lessen muscle tension, and quiet the mind. It can be done anytime, anywhere.

Time management: One of the biggest sources of stress is feeling overburdened by obligations and tasks. You can lessen emotions of overload and boost feelings of control by prioritizing activities, making a to-do list, and delegating where it's practical.

Social support: Establishing a strong support system of friends and family can give one a sense of community and lessen feelings of stress and isolation. A sounding board for challenging emotions and a sense of comfort can also be found in joining a support group or chatting to a reliable friend.

Techniques for relaxation: Yoga, tai chi, or listening to music can all be used to calm the body and mind. These methods can ease mental and physical stress and foster emotions of relaxation and tranquility.

Optimal way of life practices: Keeping a balanced diet, getting adequate sleep, abstaining from drugs, and drinking in moderation can all help to enhance general wellbeing and lessen stress. Eating well-balanced meals, getting enough rest, and abstaining from hazardous substances can all help to elevate mood, increase energy, and improve general health.

Keep in mind that every person has a unique way of dealing with stress, so what works for one person might not work for another. It's crucial to try out various methods to determine which one suits you the most, and to incorporate stress reduction into your daily routine.

Alternative Medicine for the Treatment of Heart Disease

The use of complementary or alternative therapies is an option for some people even if standard medical care is essential for managing cardiac disease. Here are a few alternative treatments for heart disease that are frequently employed:

The insertion of tiny needles into specific body locations during acupuncture therapy helps to speed up healing and lessen discomfort. By lowering stress and anxiety, enhancing circulation, and reducing inflammation, it has been used to control cardiac disease.

Yoga: This age-old discipline combines physical poses, breathing exercises, and meditation to enhance both mental and physical health. By lowering blood pressure, reducing stress and anxiety, and boosting circulation, yoga has been demonstrated to help manage cardiac disease.

herbal treatments Heart disease has long been treated with herbs like hawthorn, ginger, and garlic. Before using any herbal remedies, it's crucial to consult a doctor because some of them may interact with other prescriptions or have unwanted side effects.

massage treatment It has been demonstrated that massage therapy can assist control cardiac disease by lowering stress levels, enhancing circulation, and easing muscle tension. Additionally, it has been employed to lessen symptoms like pain, exhaustion, and anxiety.

Relaxation methods Deep breathing, meditation, and visualization exercises have all been demonstrated to improve circulation, lower blood pressure, and reduce stress—all of which are factors in the management of heart disease.

It's vital to remember that traditional medical treatment for heart disease should not be substituted with alternative remedies. Before attempting any alternative therapy, it is advisable to consult a physician to ensure that it is secure and suitable for your particular needs.

Supplements and Herbs
Numerous herbs and dietary supplements are frequently utilized for their alleged health benefits, including those for heart disease. Not all herbs and supplements, however, have been shown to be safe or helpful, and some may interact with drugs or have negative effects. Several frequently used herbs and supplements for heart health are listed below:

fatty fish: Omega-3 fatty acids, which are found in fish oil, have been demonstrated to lower inflammation and enhance heart health.

CoQ10 (coenzyme Q10): This antioxidant is essential for generating energy and is present in all body cells. Although further study is required, several studies have suggested that it might aid to enhance heart health.

Magnesium: The body needs this mineral for a variety of processes, including heart health. A higher risk of heart disease has been associated with low magnesium levels.

For its potential health benefits, especially those for heart health, garlic has been utilized for millennia. Garlic may help lower blood pressure and cholesterol levels, according to several research.

Vitamin D: Heart disease risk has been linked to low levels of vitamin D. Sunlight exposure or vitamin D pills both provide this nutrient.

Before taking any herbs or supplements, it's crucial to consult a doctor because some of them may interact negatively with prescriptions or have unwanted side effects. Supplements and herbs shouldn't be used in place of traditional medical care for heart disease.

Sure! Let me elaborate on each of these herbs and dietary supplements:

fatty fish: Omega-3 fatty acids, which are found in fish oil, have been demonstrated to provide a number of health advantages, including lowering inflammation and enhancing heart function. It is thought that omega-3 fatty acids can lower triglyceride levels, lessen the risk of blood clots, and lower the danger of heart attack and stroke.

Coenzyme Q10 (CoQ10): CoQ10 is a naturally occurring antioxidant found in every cell in the body. To assure purity and potency, it's critical to purchase a high-quality fish oil supplement that has undergone independent testing. It contributes significantly to the creation of energy and might be advantageous for heart health. Taking CoQ10 supplements may help lower blood pressure and minimize the risk of heart disease, according to several research. To fully comprehend the effects of CoQ10 on heart health, more study is necessary.

Magnesium is a vital mineral that supports the health of the heart among other biological processes. Some studies have suggested that taking magnesium supplements may assist improve heart health since low levels of magnesium have been associated to an increased risk of heart disease. To fully comprehend how magnesium affects heart health, more research is necessary.

Garlic: For millennia, people have consumed garlic because of its alleged heart-health benefits. Garlic may help lower blood pressure and cholesterol levels, both of which are risk factors for heart disease, according to some research. To completely comprehend the impact of garlic on heart health, more research is necessary.

Vitamin D is a fat-soluble vitamin that supports healthy bones, a strong immune system, and a strong heart. The risk of developing heart disease has been linked to low levels of vitamin D, and some studies have found that supplementing with vitamin

D may assist to enhance heart health. To completely comprehend the impact of vitamin D on heart health, more study is necessary.

It's crucial to keep in mind that traditional medical treatment for heart disease should not be substituted with the use of vitamins and herbs. Before using any herbs or supplements, it is always advisable to speak with a doctor because some of them may interact with certain prescriptions or have side effects. To enhance general health and wellbeing, herbs and supplements should be used in conjunction with a healthy diet and way of life.

Acupuncture

In order to promote healing and lessen pain, acupuncture is a traditional Chinese technique that involves inserting tiny needles into particular places on the body. For thousands of years, it has been used to cure a variety of illnesses, including heart disease. Using acupuncture to treat cardiac problems may do the following:

Reduces anxiety and stress: By encouraging relaxation and lowering the production of stress hormones, acupuncture can help reduce anxiety and stress. By lowering the risk of heart attack and stroke, this can promote heart health.

Circulation is improved by acupuncture, which may do so via enhancing blood flow and lowering blood pressure. By decreasing the possibility of blood clots and plaque development in the arteries, this can help lower the risk of heart disease.

Inflammation is a significant risk factor for heart disease and has been found to be reduced by acupuncture. Acupuncture may enhance heart health by lowering inflammation.

Pain relief: Acupuncture has been used to treat a variety of pain disorders, including angina, which is chest pain brought on by a decrease in the heart's blood supply.

It's crucial to remember that acupuncture shouldn't be used in place of traditional medical care for heart problems. Before considering acupuncture, it is always advisable to consult a doctor to ensure that it is both safe and suitable for your particular condition. To ensure the therapy is carried out safely and successfully, it's also crucial to select a competent and certified acupuncturist.

Yes, here is more information on the potential benefits of acupuncture for heart health:

Regulates heart rate: By enhancing the autonomic nervous system's functionality, which regulates the body's unconscious processes including heart rate and blood pressure, acupuncture may help regulate heart rate. By lowering the risk of heart attack and stroke, this can help lower the risk of developing heart disease.

Enhances cardiovascular function: By making the heart perform more efficiently and putting less strain on it, acupuncture may assist enhance cardiovascular function. By lowering the risk of heart attack and stroke, this can help lower the risk of developing heart disease.

Supports healthy lipid levels: According to certain research, acupuncture may reduce triglycerides and cholesterol, both of which are risk factors for heart disease, in order to support healthy lipid levels.

Supports healthy blood pressure: By lowering stress hormone production and encouraging relaxation, acupuncture may support healthy blood pressure. By lowering the risk of heart attack and stroke, this can help lower the risk of developing heart disease.

It's crucial to remember that acupuncture's potential advantages for treating heart disease are still being investigated, and more research is required to completely comprehend its results. However, when utilized in addition to traditional medical care, acupuncture can be a complementary therapy for controlling cardiac problems. A doctor should be consulted before beginning any complementary therapy, including acupuncture, to ensure that the treatment is safe and suitable for your particular needs.

Yoga and Meditation

Yoga is an ancient Indian physical, mental, and spiritual discipline that includes a variety of physical postures, breathing techniques, meditation, and moral and ethical principles. The ultimate goal of yoga is to achieve a condition of calmness and spiritual awareness.

In order to achieve a cognitively clear and emotionally peaceful condition, meditation includes focusing one's mind on a certain object, topic, or activity. Yoga and meditation go hand in hand rather frequently, and many spiritual traditions value meditation highly. Yoga and meditation work well together to lessen stress, enhance physical health, deepen inner calm, and advance general wellbeing.

The foundation of yoga is the idea that the mind, body, and spirit are all interrelated. Yoga has been practiced for thousands of years. The asanas, or physical poses, of yoga are intended to stretch and strengthen joints and muscles, increase circulation, and support balance and flexibility. The pranayama (breath control exercises) aid in controlling breath and calming the mind. Yoga incorporates mindfulness and meditation, which help to foster a deeper sense of awareness and inner tranquility.

Since ancient times, people have utilized meditation to calm their brains, lessen tension, and enhance their general well-being. In order to still the mind and attain a state of relaxation and mental clarity, it entails focusing one's attention on a particular thing, idea, or action, such as the breath, a mantra, or a visualization. There are many different techniques to meditate, such as sitting meditation, walking meditation, and yoga meditation.

Yoga and meditation work well together to promote physical, mental, and spiritual well-being, making this combination particularly potent. Through consistent practice, people can improve their self-awareness, lower their stress levels, sharpen their attention, and feel happier and more at peace inside. Additionally, studies have demonstrated that practicing yoga and meditation regularly can have advantageous impacts on physical health, including lowering blood pressure, enhancing sleep, and lessening anxiety and depressive symptoms.

Yoga and meditation have numerous advantages for both physical and mental health, but they are also frequently employed in spiritual contexts. Yoga is viewed by many as a means of establishing a connection with the divine and one's higher self. The ultimate aim of yoga philosophy is to liberate oneself from the cycle of birth and death and get to a state of self-realization. Additionally, meditation is thought to improve focus, self-awareness, and a deeper comprehension of reality.

People of various ages and skill levels are able to practice yoga and meditation. Yoga comes in a wide variety of forms, each with an own focus and method that makes it suitable for people of all ages and physical abilities. Similar to this, there are many different kinds of meditation, ranging from straightforward mindfulness techniques to more complex ones that include mantra repetition and visualization.

Finding a style and instructor that share your personal values and objectives is crucial. You may establish a secure and efficient practice with the assistance of a trained teacher, who can also offer direction and support as you advance. Yoga and meditation can be helpful tools for fostering general well-being, whether your goals are to enhance your physical health, lessen stress, or develop your spiritual practice.

Massage Therapy

Massage therapy is a type of manual treatment where the therapist uses pressure, friction, and other techniques on the body's muscles and soft tissues in order to relieve pain, ease tension, and boost circulation. It can be used as a therapeutic therapy for a variety of medical disorders, such as musculoskeletal injuries and chronic pain, as well as for relaxation and stress reduction. Physical therapists, chiropractors, and certified massage therapists can all provide massage therapy.

The practice of applying different techniques to the body's muscles and soft tissues is known as massage therapy. In addition to providing relaxation and stress reduction, these techniques are utilized to aid in pain relief, the release of muscle tension, and the improvement of circulation. There are numerous different massage styles, each with a distinct goal and procedure. Swedish massage, deep tissue massage, sports massage, trigger point therapy, and Shiatsu are some of the most popular massage therapy modalities. To produce the intended effects, each technique employs a different mix of pressure, friction, and other physical manipulations.

Numerous medical disorders, such as musculoskeletal injuries, chronic pain, stress, headaches, and fibromyalgia, can be treated with massage treatment. Additionally, it is frequently utilized as a therapy in addition to other medical procedures like chiropractic and physical therapy.
Physical therapists, chiropractors, and certified massage therapists all provide this service. It's critical to select a therapist with the training, experience, and expertise required to use the precise methods required to treat your unique disease.
In general, massage therapy can be a beneficial kind of treatment for many people, relieving pain, tension, and stress

while also enhancing both physical and mental health.

The various therapeutic advantages of massage treatment have been extensively acknowledged for thousands of years. Numerous health advantages can be obtained through massage treatment when carried out by a licensed therapist, including:
Releasing tight muscles, reducing muscular spasms, and relieving pain in the muscles and joints are all benefits of massage therapy.
Improved circulation can result in better overall health and a lower risk of disease since massage treatment increases blood flow to the muscles and tissues.
Reducing stress and anxiety: Studies have demonstrated that massage treatment has a relaxing effect on the mind and body, reducing tension and anxiety levels and enhancing general well-being.

Immune system stimulation: Research has revealed that massage therapy stimulates the creation of white blood cells, which are essential to the body's immune system.

Enhancing the quality of sleep: Massage therapy can aid in relaxation, which lowers the risk of sleep disorders and enhances the quality of sleep.

It's crucial to remember that massage therapy should never take the place of medical care. Before beginning massage treatment, it's crucial to speak with your healthcare provider to be sure it's safe and suitable for you if you have a medical problem.

In summary, massage therapy is a secure, non-invasive, and organic sort of treatment that can aid in enhancing both physical and emotional health. Massage therapy could be a good treatment choice for you if you want to relax, relieve tension, or both.

Role of Social Support in Managing Heart Disease

Social support plays a critical role in managing heart disease. People with a strong support system tend to have better health outcomes, including lower rates of depression, improved quality of life, and a greater ability to manage the physical and emotional demands of a chronic illness like heart disease.

Having a supportive network of friends, family, and healthcare providers can help individuals with heart disease:

- Adhere to medical regimens: Having social support can encourage individuals to follow their doctor's recommendations and take their medications as prescribed.

- Cope with emotional stress: People with heart disease often experience anxiety, depression, and other emotional stressors. Having a supportive network can help provide emotional support, decrease feelings of isolation, and improve mental health.
- Make lifestyle changes: Heart disease can often be managed through lifestyle changes, such as a healthier diet and regular exercise. Having social support can help individuals make these changes and stick to them over the long-term.
- Engage in physical activity: Social support can also help individuals with heart disease become more active. For example, joining a walking or exercise group can help individuals stay motivated and encouraged.

In addition to providing emotional support, social support can also play a critical role in providing practical assistance, such as helping with transportation to appointments or assisting with household tasks.

Overall, social support is a vital component of heart disease management, and individuals with heart disease are encouraged to build and maintain a strong support system to improve their health outcomes and quality of life.

Social support has been found to have a significant impact on the physical and mental health of individuals with heart disease. Studies have shown that people with strong social support are more likely to adhere to their medical regimen, have lower rates of depression, and have better health outcomes compared to those without strong support networks.

One of the key ways social support can help individuals with heart disease is by improving their ability to make and maintain lifestyle changes. For example, having a supportive network of friends and family members who encourage healthy eating habits, physical activity, and stress management can help individuals with heart disease make and stick to these changes over time.

Social support can also help individuals with heart disease cope with the emotional stress of living with a chronic condition. Heart disease can be a difficult and overwhelming condition, and having a supportive network of friends, family members, and healthcare providers can provide emotional support, reduce feelings of isolation, and improve overall mental health.

In addition, social support can provide practical assistance, such as helping with transportation to medical appointments or assisting with household tasks. This type of support can be especially important for individuals who have limited mobility or difficulty managing the physical demands of their condition.

Finally, participating in support groups for individuals with heart disease can also be beneficial. These groups provide a sense of community and a safe space for individuals to share their experiences, learn from one another, and receive support from others who understand the challenges of living with heart disease.

In conclusion, social support plays a critical role in the management of heart disease. By providing emotional, practical, and social support, individuals with heart disease can improve their health outcomes and quality of life.

Support Groups

People have the chance to interact with others who are going through the same struggles or experiences through support groups, a form of social support. Given that they offer a secure and encouraging environment in which people can share their experiences, thoughts, and coping mechanisms, these groups can be especially helpful for those who suffer from long-term diseases like heart disease.

A few advantages of joining a support group for people with heart disease are as follows:

Support groups give people a sense of community and a secure setting in which to discuss their feelings and experiences in relation to their illness. The group's members can provide emotional support, empathy, and understanding, which can lessen feelings of loneliness and enhance mental health.

Information and experience sharing: Support groups give people the chance to talk about their experiences, learn from one another, and get fresh perspectives and coping mechanisms connected to living with heart disease.

Encouragement and motivation: Members of support groups can offer support and motivation to one another in order to maintain medical regimens, alter lifestyles, and exercise.

Normalization of experiences: Participating in support groups gives people the chance to realize that they are not alone in their struggles and that others are going through similar things. This can lessen their sense of stigma and loneliness by normalizing their experiences.

Support groups may be led by medical professionals, neighborhood associations, or patient advocacy organizations. They can take place offline or online, and they can be professional or informal.

In summary, people with heart disease can benefit greatly from support groups. Support groups can help people with heart disease enhance their quality of life and health outcomes by offering them emotional, educational, and social support.

People with heart illness can benefit from support groups, which also provide them the chance to connect with others going through similar difficulties. An individual can obtain emotional support, share knowledge and experiences, receive inspiration and motivation, and feel as though their feelings are normalized by taking part in a support group.

One of the key advantages of support groups is the availability of emotional assistance. A secure and encouraging environment is provided by support groups for people to talk about their experiences and feelings linked to their condition. People with heart disease frequently endure emotional stress and anxiety. It can assist to lessen feelings of loneliness and enhance mental health when group members can provide empathy, understanding, and a listening ear.

Support groups give people the chance to talk about their experiences, learn from one another, and get fresh perspectives and coping mechanisms linked to living with heart disease. People can give advice on how to follow their treatment plans, alter their lifestyles, and exercise, for instance, which can be helpful for those who are finding it difficult to make these changes on their own.

Support groups can offer participants motivation and inspiration in addition to providing them with emotional and informational support. People with heart disease can feel encouraged and inspired to make improvements in their own lives by hearing about the struggles and accomplishments of others. For those who find it difficult to follow their medical regimens or alter their lifestyles, this may be of particular importance.

Last but not least, support groups provide people the chance to realize that they are not alone in their struggles and that others go through the same things. This can lessen their sense of stigma and loneliness by normalizing their experiences.

In conclusion, support groups are an important tool for people with heart disease. Support groups can assist people enhance their quality of life and health outcomes by offering emotional, educational, and social support. They provide a secure and encouraging setting where individuals can interact with others who are dealing with comparable difficulties and exchange experiences and sentiments.

Support groups can also provide people a sense of community and belonging. People who are experiencing isolation or feeling alone may find it extremely helpful to engage in meaningful relationships with people who share their experiences in support groups. People can feel more in control of their situation and positive about the future when they have a strong sense of community.

Access to a multitude of information and resources is another advantage of joining a support group. Members of the group can exchange knowledge regarding the most recent therapies, drugs, and treatments for heart disease as well as sources for symptom management and life quality enhancement. Information on nearby and online resources for people with heart disease, such as patient advocacy organizations and support programs, can also be obtained from support groups.

Last but not least, support groups can serve as a platform for activity and advocacy. Individuals with heart illness can join forces to push for improved care and treatments, participate in neighborhood activities and projects to promote heart health, and raise awareness of the problem by getting in touch with others who are going through similar struggles.

In conclusion, support groups are essential in the lives of those who have heart disease. Assistance groups can help people manage their conditions, improve their health outcomes, and lead more rewarding lives by offering them emotional, educational, social, and communal support. Consider joining a support group if you or someone you know is dealing with heart disease so you can get the help and tools you need to succeed.

The Importance of a Strong Social Network

A robust social network is crucial for controlling specific medical diseases, such as heart disease, as well as for general health and wellbeing. The connections and relationships people have with others, such as family, friends, neighbors, and community members, are referred to as social networks.

Some of the ways that people with heart disease can benefit from having a strong social network include the following:

Strong relationships with others can provide people a sense of emotional support and lessen feelings of loneliness. This is important for everyone, but it can be especially crucial for people with chronic disorders like heart disease. A robust social network can make people feel less alone and more connected, which can enhance their general mental health and well-being.

Better health habits: A strong social network can support and encourage healthy habits including regular exercise, a balanced diet, and adherence to prescribed medications. For instance, friends and family members can support and encourage people who have heart disease to make healthy lifestyle changes that will benefit their overall health.

Research has found that those with strong social networks typically experience better health results, including enhanced heart health. This is believed to be partly because social support has beneficial effects on stress levels, behavioral changes, and general health.

Access to information and resources: People with a strong social network have access to knowledge and resources that can help them manage their illness. For instance, friends and family members can connect people with various resources and support services as well as offer practical support, like providing transportation to medical appointments.

In conclusion, people with heart disease should have a robust social network. A strong social network can aid people with heart disease in managing their illness and enhancing their general health and well-being by offering emotional support, promoting healthy habits, improving health outcomes, and providing access to resources and information.

Additionally, having a supportive social network can help people manage the stress and difficulties that come with having a cardiac condition. Having a network of friends and family members who are there for you when you need them can make you feel more in control of your situation and provide you support when things go tough.

Furthermore, people with heart disease can keep their independence and stay active with the aid of a strong social network. For instance, friends and family members can offer chances for people to take part in social events, neighborhood activities, and other hobbies, preventing social isolation and enhancing general wellbeing.

The sharing of knowledge and information is a key component of a robust social network. People with heart disease can learn about new treatments, drugs, and therapies as well as get guidance and suggestions for managing their illness by interacting with others who are going through similar struggles. They can also impart their own wisdom and experiences, which will be helpful to the group as a whole.

Last but not least, having a strong social network can give you a feeling of direction and significance. People with heart disease might feel more a part of something bigger than themselves by engaging in social activities, giving back to the community, and making connections with people who have similar interests. This can enhance their feeling of overall wellbeing.

In conclusion, people with heart disease need to have strong social networks. A strong social network can help people with heart disease live full, meaningful lives despite their condition by offering emotional support, encouraging good habits, improving health outcomes, providing access to services and information, and increasing involvement.

Developing Bonds with Healthcare Professionals

For people with heart disease, developing close relationships with medical professionals is crucial because it can enhance overall quality of life and health outcomes. The following are some pointers for creating enduring connections with medical professionals:

Any strong relationship, including those with healthcare providers, is built on good communication. People should feel at ease communicating their questions, worries, and information to their healthcare professional.

To get the most out of each appointment with a healthcare professional, preparation is essential. People should be ready with a list of queries, worries, and any updates on their health, such as adjustments to their medication or changes in symptoms.

Participate actively in your own care: Patients should actively participate in their own care by pursuing suggested therapies, raising concerns with their doctor about their progress, and asking questions.

Trust: A crucial component of any connection, including ones with healthcare professionals, is trust. People should have faith in their healthcare professional to deliver the finest care possible and be prepared to heed their advice.

Find a service provider you are at ease with: People should feel at ease with their healthcare practitioner, and if they don't, they should think about finding another one who will make them feel more at ease.

Regular check-ins with medical professionals can help sustain the relationship and guarantee that patients receive the treatment they require.

In conclusion, people with heart disease must establish trusting relationships with their medical professionals. People can enhance their health outcomes and general quality of life by establishing open communication, being an active participant in their treatment, developing trust, finding a physician they are comfortable with, and having regular check-ins.

expand

Better health results might also result from a close relationship with a healthcare professional. For instance, a clinician who is aware of a patient's health background, way of life, and preferences might modify advice and treatments to better suit that patient's requirements.

Additionally, adherence to treatment plans can be enhanced by having a solid relationship with a healthcare professional. People are more likely to adhere to suggested treatments, take medications as directed, and adopt lifestyle changes that can improve their health when they feel at ease and trust their provider.

Additionally, the worry and anxiety that come with managing a chronic condition like heart disease can be lessened by establishing a close relationship with a healthcare professional. People are more likely to feel secure and less overwhelmed by their condition when they believe that their provider understands their requirements and is available to support them.

Last but not least, having a solid relationship with a healthcare professional can give people access to the most recent data and tools for controlling heart disease. In addition to providing referrals to specialists and other healthcare professionals when needed, providers can provide information on fresh therapies, drugs, and treatments.

In conclusion, maintaining close contact with a healthcare professional is crucial for managing heart disease. A solid relationship with a healthcare professional can help people with heart disease lead better, more happy lives by encouraging open communication, encouraging adherence to treatment programs, lowering stress and anxiety, and offering access to resources and information.

Summary of Natural Solutions for Managing Heart Disease

There are a number of all-natural ways to treat heart disease, including:

Exercise: Regular physical activity can help to improve cardiovascular health and lower the risk of heart disease, making it a crucial component of managing heart disease.

Eating well: Eating a diet high in fruits, vegetables, whole grains, and lean proteins can help control heart disease and enhance heart health.

Stress management: By lowering blood pressure, increasing heart rate, and reducing inflammation, managing stress can help lower the risk of heart disease. Stress management techniques including deep breathing, meditation, and yoga can be beneficial.

Quit smoking: Smoking is a significant risk factor for heart disease, so giving up can help lower that risk and enhance general health.

Sleep: Getting adequate good sleep is crucial for maintaining heart health since it helps lower blood pressure, improve heart rate, and help people feel less stressed.

Weight control: Keeping a healthy weight helps lower your risk of developing heart disease because being overweight places more strain on your heart.

Supplements: A number of supplements, including fish oil, magnesium, and vitamin D, can assist to strengthen the heart and lower the chance of developing heart disease.

In conclusion, these herbal remedies can help manage heart disease and enhance general health when combined with medical therapies and lifestyle modifications. Before beginning any new natural remedies, it's crucial to speak with a doctor, though, as some supplements may interact with prescription drugs and other treatments.